Content

Acknowledgment

My big thanks to Dina Zalizniak – talented painter and creator of all those beautiful pictures which you can see in this book.

Also my deep appreciation to all who reviewed this book and did lots useful remarks and advises regarding correct languages and over-whole book understanding.

Regards to everybody who helps me to become better and more conscious through lots of negotiations and exercises.

Thank you much all!

About the author

Author of this small book is an ordinary man. Let me say not high, not low. He has the same pros and cons like all others. He likes good food, nice friendly atmosphere, good weather, travels, interesting book, cinema etc. His hobby and his work - network systems design. Been born in Ukraine, at the moment author works as a System Security Engineer for semi-government entity in UAE. He is engaged in systems design and deployment of IP video surveillance, networking, virtualization of data centers. He is expat and at the moment live and work in United Arab Emirates.

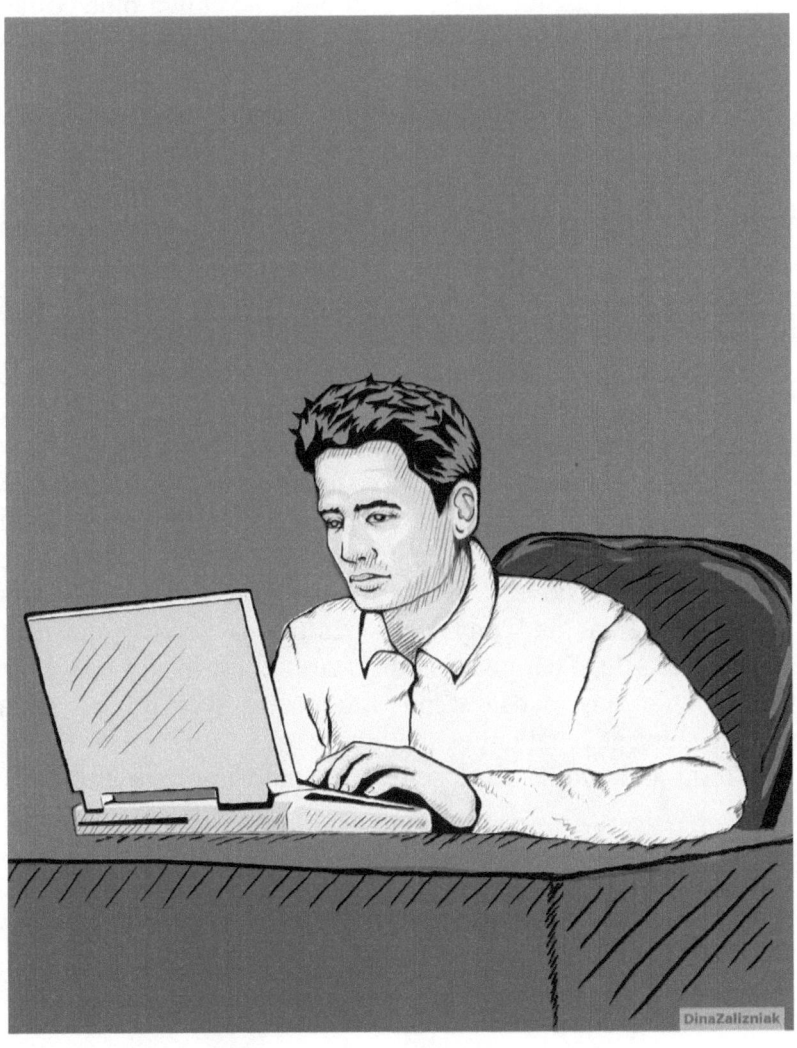

Introduction

Let me say from beginning – you can do it! You are not worse than others. Yeas, you are busy, tired, overwhelmed with regular tasks and works. This is your life. But you can. Less think – just do. Start to change your life right now. Burn your fat, reduce weight not tomorrow or from beginning of the month, but now. Stand up and make first step.

It is seems a bit strange that this book written by Network Engineer – profession which very far from fitness, bodybuilding or sport at all. On other hand, such approach allows to look at diet subject from completely different point of view. Through eyes of millions field engineers, office clerks, technicians and other so called blue collar staff. I am one of them. Always busy, always loaded with hundred tasks. But I did it. I succeed. Why you can not?

In my case everything began with simple football game. My colleagues play football 2 -3 times per week. Many company staff participate in that game. And me too. My first game was awful. After first part I was completely exhausted. My legs not moved. My team was angry with me and I was forced to leave the field after first part. I was upset. I never expected to bee so weak. But what I should expect if I did not participate in any sport activities for years ? Overwhelmed by those unhappy thoughts I spent few days in bad mood. One day, on my way home, I saw lighted windows of small gym. And suddenly something inside me said - "let's come and ask. Why not ?". That visit changed my life. I started regularly visit the gym . But it changed my life even more when I started to read and listen more about exercises and sport nutrition. My wish to improve sport results suddenly led me to unexpected conclusions. I find out, that first and foremost way to improve your mental and physical health is healthy nutrition and proper day schedule. That conclusion changed lot in my life. It did not removed my everyday loads but give me more power, force and stamina to pass all current challenges. I was really surprise how simple, everyday food and proper time schedule could improve and bright my life.

A bit of theory

So let me also try to improve your live and share my knowledge, my experience with you. First of all we should more-less clear understand our task and goals, theoretical and practical parts.

In order to understand how to burn excessive fat let's briefly have a look at what it is - "FAT"

First of all - "Fat" - it is also nutrition reserve of our body. And let me note, that body does not like to be feed from that reserve. There few different types of the fat inside us . Mainly there 4 types of fat in our body:

- White fat. Formed by white adipocytes. Involved in energy accumulation and hormone production. Typical value in a body - 15—25% ;

- Brown fat. Mainly responsible for energy spending. Formed with vessels and glands and has relation to mitochondrias. Mainly located near kidney, back, shoulders, neck. Typical value in a body - less than 5%;

- Beige fat. Unique type of cells . Could be converted to White fat or to Brown fat under influence of stress conditions;

- Subcutaneous fat. Located just under skin of a human. Protect body from over cooling. Accumulates energy. Considered as hormone active tissue. The accumulation of subcutaneous fat depends on gender (in women is always greater than in men), on age (increases with medium age, decreases in old age) and dietary habits (increases with physical inactivity and overeating). Typical value in a body - up to 90% ;

-Visceral fat. Most dangerous type of the fat. Visceral fat is white fat that is found in the abdominal cavity around organs, liver, pancreas, heart, intestines. Researchers have found that visceral fat secretes retinol-binding protein 4, which increases insulin resistance. This, in turn, leads to glucose intolerance and type 2 diabetes. To estimate the amount of visceral fat in the body, you need to determine the ratio of waist to hips. Measure the waist and hips at the widest point. Then divide the waist circumference by hips circumference. If the number is greater than 1.0 in men and 0.85 in women, then the level of fat is too high.

There are few approaches and technique how to regulate different fat in our body. Mainly we should concentrate our attention on most dangerous visceral fat and that is what we will discuss in the following topics.

A bit of practice

First of all we need to remember and understand few key factors about fat, nutrition and energy. Especially energy. Energy – key to everything. If we want to burn fat and lose our weight, we must receive less energy than spend. Everyday we must receive from food less Kcall than spend during day activities.

 Our bodies love everything that gives it lot of cheap energy (chocolate, fatty food etc). And vise versa - our bodies do not love everything that leads to extra energy spending. That is why for us more pleasure to sit instead of stand, to lie instead to sit. Our brain spend nearly 25% of energy when works at full load! That is why for us more pleasure to watch light movie than complicated educational program. Comics and comedy much preferable before scientific documentary movie.

Let me note also - it is not proved that we can burn fat locally. Fat burning starts under influence of stress hormones. Those hormones freely circulate in our blood through all our body, not only in some particular part. Until we create conditions for burning fat through right diet - we can not burn it locally or burn it at all. That is why I have a quite skeptical attitude to those who promise to burn your fat abdomen locally and just in 1-2 weeks without any effort and diet :)

Ok. After brief overview of fat burn issue, let's look at some practical approaches.

Brief and straight. Just fact and some conclusions:

-To burn fat and start loosing weight we need to receive less energy than spend. It could be done in two ways – less receive (diet) or more spent (basic expenditures, sport/physical activities);

 -Diet is most important in this way as it is allows faster, easy and more accurate limits energy income;

-Physical activities, sport allows us increase energy spending. There 2 different type of physical activities – so called basic activities and heavy physical activities or sport. Basic activities -that is what our body doing when doing nothing. Means idle. To that activities belongs all processes in our body. Everything what has happened when we siting, watching TV, eating, sleeping. It is basic energy consumption. Heavy physical activities or sport that is when we are doing exercises, carrying heavy loads, doing squats or running. Or event heavy thinking. Let's note that our brain during it's hard work consume up to 25% of our energy ! So small organ but so energy consuming !;

-Do not force fat burn process as it could makes harm yourself. Very often peoples do not want to see their fatness for years. They live over-weighted, suffer from different diseases related to that. But when it comes to fat burning they try to solve all their weight related problems very fast, in emergency mode. It is not possible to solve in one day what was accumulated during many years;

-There are different medicines for speed up fat burning process. But I recommend to keep natural way. At last use a cap of strong coffee before exercises. Its natural and allows you to avoid heavy excessive medicines.

My approach and experience

What I think and what I did. I kept a diet. Diet means strict keeping chosen amount of food per day. Not only exclude some type of food. For example we could exclude all fatty food but consume even more calories from other type of nutrition (like potatoes, meat or bread for example). In this case we even increase our weight instead of reduce it.

It is recommended to eat often but small portions. I agree. It works. Such approach allows to speed-up metabolism in our bodies, improve food digesting and energy extraction. During our diet it allows also to "cheat" body and feel well fed even with less amount of food during day, that in consequence creates necessary lack of calories.

When I started my diet, I chose suitable products, chose suitable amount of those products and start to eat the same everyday. It was my Starting Point. After 2 first weeks I corrected amount (and even increased a bit). Based on my knowledge and experience, I could provide you some general recommendation for diet:
-Reduce fried and fatty food;
- Reduce fast hydro-carbonates (chocolate, sugar, sweet candies);
- Increase protein (especially animal protein) and cellular tissue (vegetables)
Meanwhile cellular tissue (vegetables) slow down digesting and transforming for hydro-carbonates and lead to better diet effect. Protein (especially animal protein) helps to save your muscles (otherwise body starts "eating" them, burning your muscles fast);
-In first 1-2 weeks your body "burns" everything that can be "burnt" first, like short hydro-carbonates and glycogen. So not be afraid to lose

about 2-4 kg for the first time. Than loses should stabilize to 0.5 -1 kg per week;

-Always eat vegetables (except before sleep). Vegetables contain cellulose that is useful for digesting;

-Take a few sugar of something sweet before work-out in a gym. Carbohydrates required for proper brain functioning. But not to much sweets. Less carbohydrates you took before gym workout – more fat you can burn;

-Carbohydrates in the morning. Protein in the evening. Simple.

Practically, very convenience to cook food for one or few day in advance. It is easy and definitely saves time. You just put ready food to your bag at the morning and go to work. Divide all food to 4 pieces and put it to 4 plastic food containers. It is better to take food in small portions but often. In such case we cheat our body a bit :) It start to think that food constantly available. You will feel not so hungry and be able to keep the diet. Take food at last 4 times per day:

    A. Morning

    B. Lunch

    C. Just after come back from work

    D. Before go to bed (low fat Cottage cheese or Casein)

As I said, low fat Cottage cheese and caw milk is very important and useful. But if your body does not accept lactose – you could use sport nutrition such as Casein (Optimum Nutrition Gold standard Casein for example). During a day drink lot of water - it speeds up metabolisms. If you need to increase or decrease energy Kcall per day – do it by means of complex hydro-carbonates (less/more Rice, Buckwheat etc.) but leave proteins.

Step-by-step program

I hope you read carefully previous chapters and now you are ready to start. In order to achieve desired results, I recommend to follow below simple program and activities:

1. Take paper notebook
   A) Write your diet start date;
   B) Write your weight;
   C) Write sizes of your belly, chest, biceps

2. Choose your preferred food for diet

   A) For example we chose: White Rice, Chicken Breast, Egg, Laban, Vegetables, Fruits;
   B)   Calculate approximately required amount of above food in accordance with my advises (and/or) nutrition table;
   C) Follow the cornerstone principals.   When start, choose suitable products, choose suitable amount of those products and start to eat the same everyday. It is your Starting Point. After 1-2 first weeks need to correct amount (increase or decrease depending on your results).

For example, for man 85 kg we are going to use:

Man's everyday diet products (approximate calculation):
-*Cup of rice (200 g) = 152 g of carbohydrates + 690 Kcal;*
-*Chicken breast (500 g)=100g of protein + 600 Kcal;*
-*Egg whites (without yolks) 7pc = 40g of protein + 154 Kcal;*
-*Whole egg (with yolk) 3pc = 27g of protein + 330 Kcal;*
-*Cottage cheese (200g low fat) = 36g of protein + 192 Kcal;*
-*Vegetables 300-500g (cucumbers, tomato, salad) = 15-20 of carbohydrates + 70-100 Kcal*

Total: approximately 2060 Kcal (170g of carbohydrates + 200g of protein)

Or
Man's everyday diet products (approximate calculation):
-*White Rice (200 g) = 152g of carbohydrates + 690 Kcal;*

-Chicken breast (500 g)=100g of protein + 600 Kcal;
-Whole egg (with yolk) 4pc = 36g of protein + 440 Kcal;
-Laban (180 ml) 3pc = 9g of protein + 180 Kcal;
-Banan 1pc = 40g of carbohydrates + 80 Kcal;
-Vegetables 300-500g (cucumbers, tomato, salad) = 15-20 of carbohydrates + 70-100 Kcal

Total: approximately - 2090 Kcall (212g of carbohydrates + 145g of protein)

If you are big person and your mass more than 90 kg, just increase your portions to achieve 2500 Kcal for beginning
Approximately energy consumption looks like this:
Man under 80 kg about 2000 Kcal;
Man above 80 kg about 2500 Kcal;

For women the same algorithm but need to reduce starting amount of calories. Women's body has less muscles than a men's. Women's body constructed by nature mainly for baby borning. That is why it loves to do emergency reserves in case of cold, hunger and other unpredictable situations.

For women to achieve required diet results it is necessary to reduce receiving calories more than for men. Very often, required lack of calories for women is something around 1000 -1500 Kcal (usually we are talking about height less 170 cm). Even regardless of her weight (weight more than 80 kg says about overweight and presence lots of fat, not muscles)
Here some advises for women:
 - You could change food in accordance with your preferences (chicken to fish, rice to buckwheat etc.). Again, the main idea – strictly follow chosen diet food and it's amount per day;
- All diet's requirements should be strictly followed. Not allowed to eat anything extra or beyond above list as it shifts your starting point;
 -May be staring point is too much high or to much lower exactly for you. In such case you should correct it slightly. You should feel light hunger during a day and be energetic and fresh. Try to catch that feeling of "light hunger" and your fat burning proceeds successfully and fast;
- Put yourself on scale every week. For women fat burning process flows slower than for men. Even if you lose 0.5 kg fat per week it is

good. If it 1 kg per week – great. But no more as you cold make harm yourself as I wrote before in this book;
- Make correction for monthlies. During this period woman's body accumulate resources for possible baby born and blood loses. It is normal to increase about 2 kg weight during that period. Usually everything return back to previous state in a few days after the monthlies. You could also decrease calories consumption before that period as physical activities during that time typically also decreases.

For example, for woman 65 kg we are going to use:

Women's everyday diet products (approximate calculation):
 -Cup of rice (100 g) = 76 g of carbohydrates + 345 Kcal
 -Chicken breast (400 g)=80 g of protein + 480Kcal
 -Egg whites (without yolks) 5pc = 28g of protein + 110 Kcal
 -Whole egg (with yolk) 3pc = 27g of protein + 330 Kcal

 -Cottage cheese (200g low fat) = 36g of protein + 192 Kcal
 -Vegetables 300-500g (cucumbers, tomato, salad) = 15-20 of carbohydrates + 70-100 Kcal

Total: approximately 1500 Kcal (100g of carbohydrates + 170g of protein)

Or
Women's everyday diet products (approximate calculation):
- *White Rice (100 g) = 76g of carbohydrates + 345 Kcal*
 -Chicken breast (500 g)=100g of protein + 600Kcal
 -Whole egg (with yolk) 3pc = 9g of protein + 330 Kcal
- *Laban (180 ml) 2pc = 6g of protein + 120 Kcal;*
 -Vegetables 300-500g (cucumbers, tomato, salad) = 15-20 of carbohydrates + 70-100 Kcal

Total: approximately - 1500 Kcall (96g of carbohydrates + 115g of protein)

Approximately energy consumption looks like this:
Woman under 60 kg about 1500 Kcal

3. Cook White Rice, Chicken, Eggs. All boiled or steamed;

4. Divide all that food by 4 pieces and put them to 4 different plastic/glass containers;

5. Write on each container: Breakfast, Lunch, Second Lunch, Dinner;

6. Schedule most convenience time when you could eat food from each container
For example: Breakfast – 08.00 when you have 15 min for break at work;

Lunch – 14.00 when you have 15 min for break at work;
Second Lunch – 19.00 just after come home from work;
Dinner – 22.00-23.00 one hour before bed;

7. **Follow this schedule – no more no less.**
Eat that set of products everyday. The same kind of food, the same amount. Change nothing.   Again - everyday the same amount and the same food
After one week:
B) Check and write down your weight;
C) Check and write down sizes of your belly, chest, biceps

8. Human body is inert and require time to adapt. That is such as heavy truck – very hard to start move and very hard to stop. But when it is run – it is run fast and stable. After one week you should see some small changes. Very carefully write them down. After 2 weeks result should be more accurate and stable;

9. Check all those changes:
- If you increase in weight – reduce amount of food by 25%;
- If you stay the same - reduce amount of food by 15%;
- If you lose weight 0.5kg -1 kg - stay the same amount. You are on right way.

N*B*
*Change all food to dietary. No fried. Only steamed or boiled.
**Please pay attention. I stress again - you should not lose more than 1 kg per/week.
If you lose more than 1 kg per week it means that your internal organs, your muscles decrease, and your health could suffer. Meanwhile losing weight too fast could lead to other effect – slow down your

metabolisms and decrease speed of your fat and weight lose. It is known as self defending reaction of your body. Body sees that something dangerous happening and tries to save itself from the death. So, stay in the limits. Control your fat and weight and not allow yourself to lose them too fast. Proper diet maintenance and regular control will lead you to success.

*** Also I need to stress some known behavior of our body during adaptation time. First week you could lose more than 1 kg – may be up to 3-4 kg. That is OK. It is possible as our body tries to manage unexpected reduce in energy income. That is why more accurate results could be achieved approximately after 2 weeks from beginning of your diet.

Sport activities

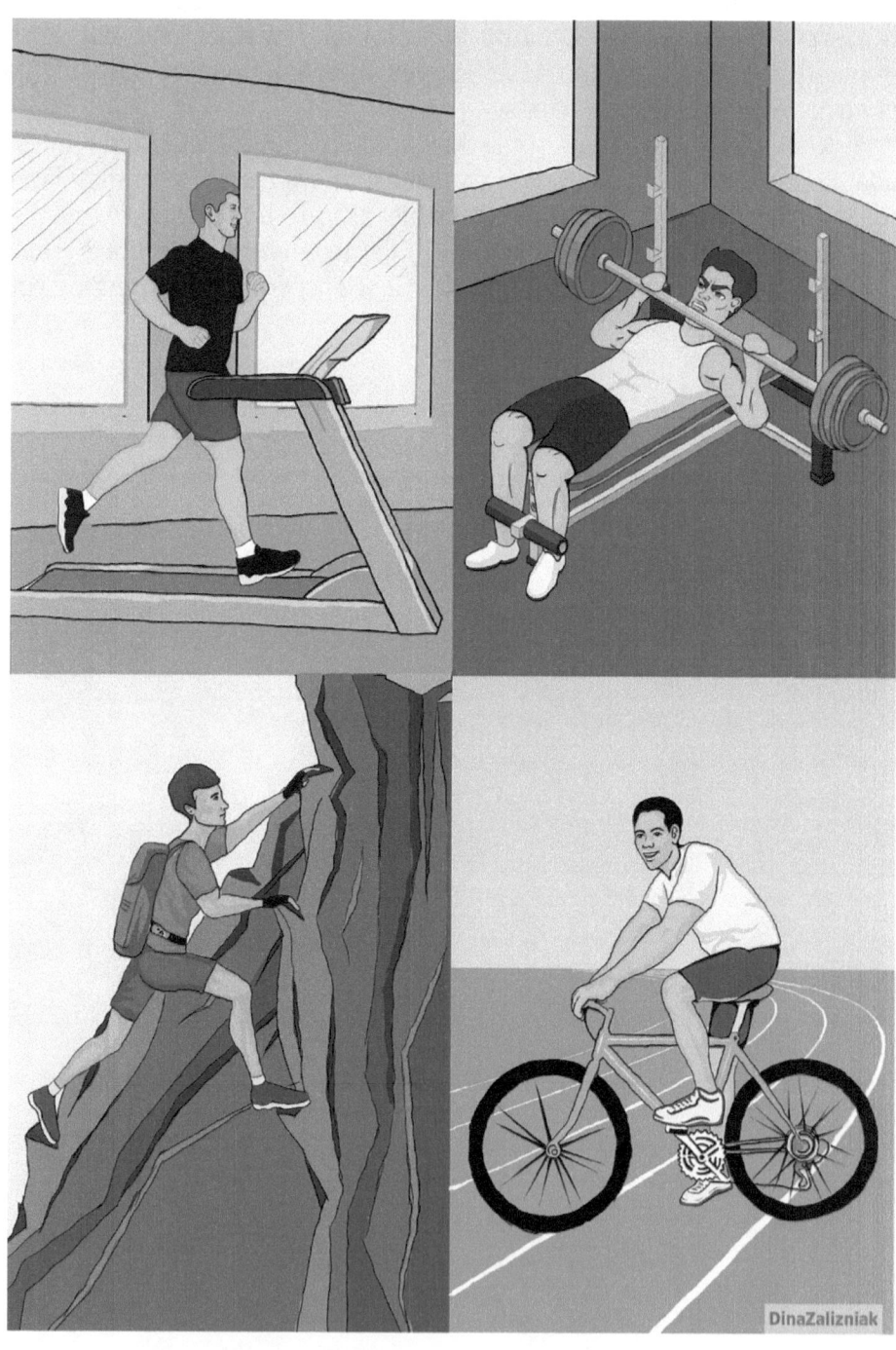

Sport and different physical exercises definitely could help us looks better, healthier and play synergistic effect with proper diet. Below are some facts and advises regrading sport and indoor/outdoor activities.

Types of physical activities:

-Aerobic activities (Cardio or running) or Anaerobic activities (training with "iron" in a gym);

-Aerobic activity more energy consuming and uses fat as main energy source *just in the process*, during training. Affects fat burning right during exercises;

-Anaerobic activity (training with "iron" in a gym) creates bigger deficit of calories *after* training. And that deficit is really bigger than it is during Aerobic activities if we consider 24 hour period;

-Worth to mention that during deficit of calories, body starts to "eat" your muscles, not fat only. And Anaerobic activity (training with "iron" in a gym) prevent this as force muscles to work.

Meanwhile, one more issue related to insulin resistance – Anaerobic activities increase cells' sensitivity to insulin and helps such people start burn fat (in fatty people cells' insulin sensitivity reduced, that leads to getting fatty even more);

-Conclusion regarding activities – first place an Anaerobic activity (training with "iron" in a gym), second Aerobic activities (Cardio or running). The best solution is to combine both types of activities (Aerobic activity in the morning + Anaerobic activity in the evening for example);

-The main goal of an Anaerobic activity (training with "iron" in a gym) is to save muscles but not burn them like a firewood!;

-Long cyclic load uses fat as a source of energy. The core of this activity are periodic, long term (15min -2hours) repeating actions with low intensity (like walking, slow running, rowing, cycling, etc.). When a load is so small that does not require much energy at once, body prefers to extract energy from the fat. It is very important – intensity should be low, otherwise in a lack of energy body starts to extract it from carbohydrates instead of the fat. Conclusion: Aerobic activities (Cardio or walking) should be long enough but not intensive. To burn just fat we should walk (actually not run), but walk long as 1hour – 2 hours end even more;

-Aerobic and Anaerobic activities both are very useful to effectively burn fat;

-Aerobic activities should be low intensive and long lasting (running or walking slowly for more than one hour – use player and headset – great opportunities to listen to your lovely audio book!);

-Aerobic activities, performed with low intensities and long lasting, burns fat directly, not consuming glycogen or other "fast" energy resources;

-Anaerobic activities burns "fast" energy resources first (like glycogen) and less related to fat burning, but it exhausts organism more than - Aerobic activities. If we look at 24hour scale, Anaerobic activities lead to grater energy spending per that period. That is why recommended workout in a gym;

-Anaerobic activities also stabilize insulin level in our blood that allow us more effective proceed with diet.

So, as it was mentioned - the best solution is to combine both types of activities (Aerobic activity in the morning + Anaerobic activity at night for example). All those combinations has advantages and disadvantages. Brief summaries regarding Aerobic activities (Cardio or walking):

-    Exercises at *morning*, before breakfast. This time of lack of hydro-carbonates - Most effective but also most harmful for your muscles as it burns them very fast. In this case recommended to use some kind of sport nutrition, called BCAA that helps a bit to save your muscles;

- Exercises *after Anaerobic* activity (training with "iron" in a gym). Effective method as your muscles already burnt hydro-carbonates during training and now body starts to extract energy from the fat;

- Exercises *before sleep*. Also effective time for Aerobic activities. As we eat only protein before sleep, this method creates lack of hydro-carbonates for all night and force body to use fat as an energy.

Typical recommended scheme for sport activities during diet:

Choice 1

-Morning – slowly running or walking more that 60 min;
-Evening – workout in a gym for 60 min;

Choice 2

- Evening – workout in a gym 60 min + slow running or walking 60 min;

We also should remember that muscles are big energy accumulators and the same time big energy consumers. More muscles we have - more energy we could accumulate and spent during a period of time. That is why it is much easy to burn fat for people who have bigger muscles. But every exercises for muscles first of all lead to their grow (anabolism), not to decrease (catabolism). So, training abdomen area leads to muscles grow in that place and your waist getting thicker (not thinner). Sure, you should do exercises for you waist but to remove extra fat from there you should keep the diet.

Healthy nutrition

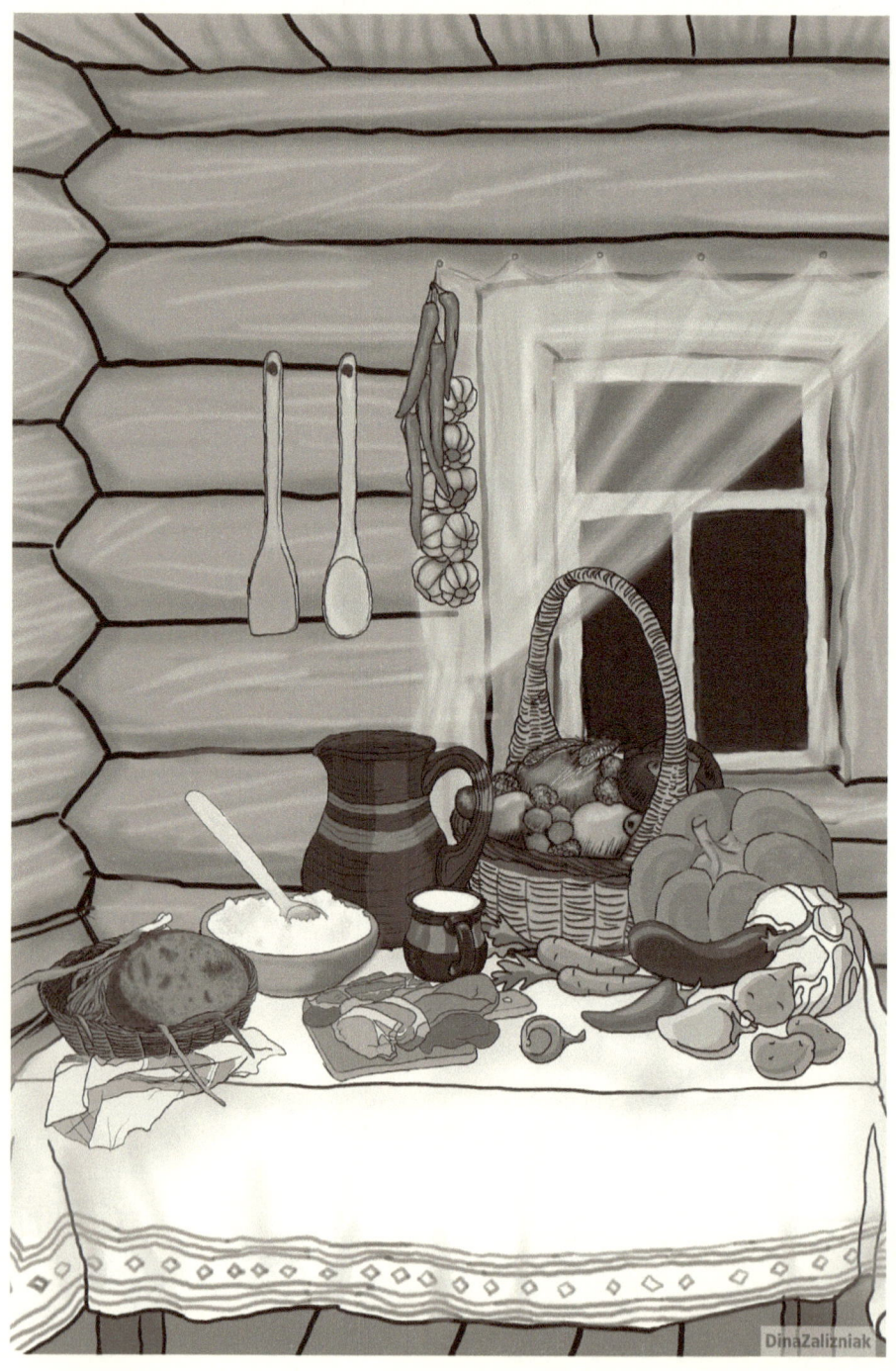

It was in 1826 that French physician and Godfather of the low-carb diets Jean Anthelme Brillat-Savarin wrote: Dis-moi ce que tumanges, je te dirai ce que tu es. "Tell me what you eat, and I will tell you what you are."

I could agree with this saying. The good things that gym gave me - are the proper nutrition habits.
Really, nearly all of us busy, from delivery guy, cycling all day by city streets to top manager, who could sits under papers 12-14 hours in his office. But all of us are humans. I have simple, "mechanical" approach to this issue. As our cars required fuel (any type), - our body require food to support our lives. And it is common for anybody – poor man or millionaire.

Rhythm of life put it's fingertips on our nutrition habits. Before I even did not think under it. I ate anything, anywhere, anytime. As a result – problem with health, tooth illness, stomach pain and gases, irregular and anxious sleep. And this is even not all :). I am not saying about weak muscles and pear-shape body. I think many of you recognize yourself from this characteristics.

As I mentioned everything changed when I went to gym. But mainly not because the exercises.
Because I stared to read about athletes' food. Listen different broadcast, dedicated to sport, anatomy and food industry. And find out that eat healthy quit simple. No need to spend lot's of money for private cook or going every time to restaurant. Through obtained knowledge and my personal experience I created a list of simple and not expansive household appliances and products that you could use in your everyday life. Usually I have no much time for cooking and I follow practical approach to food. Food should be healthy, natural, maximum effective. It should not take much time for cooking. It is should be easy to cook and preserve in a fridge for few days.

Based on above reasoning I could advise you to pay your attention to the next:

List of machines and mechanisms for your kitchen:
-Steam cooker;
-Electrical induction stove;
-Microwave;
-Kettle;
-Fridge;
-Regular household appliances

List of food products which should be in your ration:
-Chicken breast, Beef, Fish;
-Egg;
-White cow cheese (low fat), Milk, Yogurt, Laban;
-Buckwheat, White Rice, Millet, Semolina;
-Vegetables, Fruits;

As we are human, men and women from bones and blood – we should eat. Food gives us power and will to live. But somebody live to eat and somebody eat to live. Feel the difference! I keep the second part of statement – I eat to live. From this point of view, I think food should be maximally practical, fast cooking and effective.
Below some useful and practical advises regarding the types of food and how it could be cooked.

White Rice

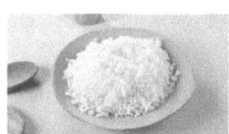

Universal source of long "slow" carob-hydrates. Depending on type of your diets (weight loss or mass grow) you could prepare different amount of this product. Rice makes stronger your stomach, covering it by thing film from inside. You could could cook about 400 g (in raw) of white rice and leave it in fridge for 2 days. Rice is nice to eat with fish, meat (beef, chicken), vegetable, BBQ. You could eat rice with milk and sugar. Cook rice very easy (one from many receipts). Put 400 gr of white rice to the can. Wash it in cold water 3 times. Then place the can on stove. Wait until water is boiling and cook till rice becomes soft (approximately 10-15 min). Remove from stove and pour out to sieve. Wait until rice get cool. It is ready. Rice could be served as garnish with chicken, beef, mushrooms etc. Also possible to eat rice with milk and sugar. This is good, healthy product which allows you always be well fed. And it is easy with rice to regulate amount of income energy (Kcal). Spend 20 minutes and you will have guaranteed source of "slowly" carbohydrates for 2 days.

Buckwheat

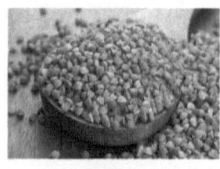

Universal source of long "slow" carbohydrates. Depending on type of your diets (weight loss or grow) you could prepare different amount of this product. Just put one glass 200 gr of dry Buckwheat to can, add 3 glass of water and wait until it is boiling. Than add 2 big spoon of sunflower oil, reduce stove temperature and cook until all water evaporated. It is ready. Could be served with different types of meat, fish, sauce or just eat it with milk and sugar. Very universal and effective nutrition.

Millet

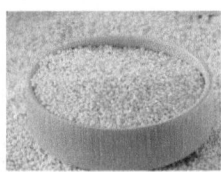

Similar to Buckwheat, Millet is universal source of long "slow" carbohydrates. Depending on type of your diets (weight loss or grow) you could prepare different amount of this product. Just put one glass 200 gr of dry Millet to can, add 3 glass of water and wait until it is boiling. Than add 2 big spoon of sunflower oil, reduce stove temperature and cook until all water evaporated. It is ready. Could be served with different types of meat, fish, sauce or just eat it with milk and sugar. Very universal and effective nutrition. More recipes you could find online. Millet could be easy saved in a fridge up to 1 week!

Semolina

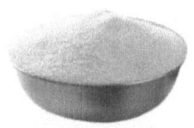

The easiest and fastest to prepare natural source of protein. Firstly, semolina it is a source of protein, with almost 6 grams per serving! It is also rich in B vitamins, including folate and thiamine, which help create energy and support brain function. Selenium is another benefit to semolina, one that serves as an antioxidant to help prevent heart disease! Just heat nearly to boil 0.5 of milk, add 4 dining spoon of Semolina, a bit raisins for flavor, mix it all well when heating 2-3 min and healthy dish ready!

White cow cheese (low fat)

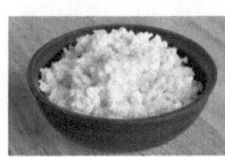

Unique source of proteins. So called long-digesting proteins. Naturally could replace know sport additive as Casein. Take 250 gr of *White cow cheese 0.5% fat*, add low fat sour cream and one big spoon of honey. Excellent, testy nutrition. Eat every evening before sleep. Your body digest it slowly and will be well fed with proteins and vitamins during night.

Laban(Leben (milk product))

Laban refers to a food or beverage of fermented milk. Generally, there are two main products known as leben: in

the Levant region, yogurt; and in Arabia and North Africa (Maghreb), buttermilk. The practice of intentionally allowing milk to sour has been known since ancient times and practiced by many cultures. Rich of vitamins and useful bacteria. Helps digest food faster. Laban is a fermented milk product that is produced by bacterial fermentation of milk and it is little thick and creamy. Our body needs a few amount of "good" bacteria in the digestive part and the Laban contains "good" bacteria. Laban or low fat Yogurt/Yoghurt is easily digested and less lactose than milk and it is good for bones, boost immune system and helps to make soft skin. It is highly nutritious and also a good source of protein, calcium, vitamins, etc. It will reduce the risk of diseases like high blood pressure, Colon Cancer, Diarrhea and heart diseases.

Chicken Breast

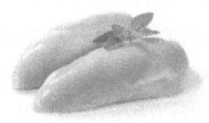
"Foundation" of everyday food. It is as for weight grow, as for diet for fat burn and weight lost. Just use various amount. Very fast to cook. Tasty and useful. Not expensive. Available everywhere. You could cook Chicken Breast in different ways. But I recommend cook it on steam or boil. For example, take 500 gr fresh or unfrozen chicken breast. Cut it in peaces of medium size, put them to steam cooker. Add grated carrot, onion, tomato and eggplant. Cook for 20-30 min (steam cooker often has it's own mode for "Steam" - 20 min for example). Or take 500 gr fresh chicken breast. Put to a can. Add one liter of water. Add small grated carrot, pepper peas, bay leaf, few pieces of garlic. Boil it 25-30 min. At the end you will get very testy, powerful soup which will recover your strength in a minutes and allow to feel good no less a half of the day.

Beef

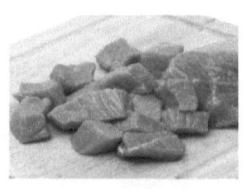
As we, know, the best amino-acid composition we could get only if we are eating different food. To complete this requirements and complete our nutrition balance, we should include to our ration

different types of meat. Beef is a good choice. Not fat, reach of protein and required amino-acids.

Here it is one of the way to cook it fast and effective. Take 500 g of fresh or unfrozen beef. Slice it. Prepare cream sauce and keep sliced pieces of beef in it about 1 hour or more. After that put sliced pieces of beef to steam cooker. Add grated carrot and put on each sliced beef 2 piece of pineapple. Cook 20-25 min. Very tasty, healthy and useful dish!

Eggs

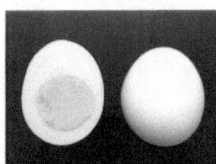 Eggs are also "Foundation" of everyday food. During fat and weight lost it is recommended to eat Eggs without yolk. For weight grow you could include at least 4 whole eggs with yolk per day. Egg could be taken as standard of nutrition. As it has 100% balanced ratio of all required nutrition elements. It is easy to boil egg and keep them for 2-3 days in a fridge. Just take can, put 12 eggs, add water that it cover all eggs. A bit salt. And keep boiling 10 min. After that drain hot water and replace it with cold water. Wait until all eggs is cool. Perfect food for everyday. You could take it with you to office or to workshop, to any place where your work.

Vegetables

Vegetables – great source of cellulose and vitamins. During diet you should include vegetables. If it possible – you could eat nearly unlimited amount of vegetables. Vegetables allow your stomach functioning better. Tomatoes, onion, carrot, cucumber, spinach, cabbage will make your food reach of vitamin, effective and very useful.

Fruits

Fruits – great source of cellulose and vitamins. But some of them holds a lot of sugars or calories. So be careful when include them in everyday ration. Refer to Nutrition Values tables or online sources.

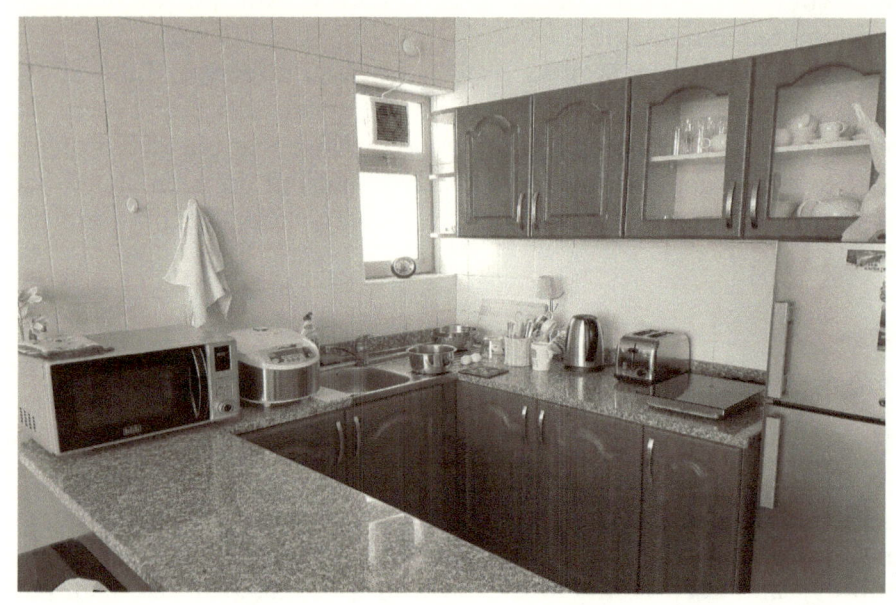

My kitchen. Simple and effective.

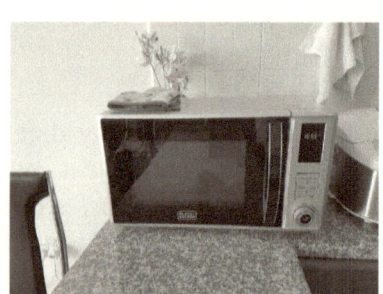
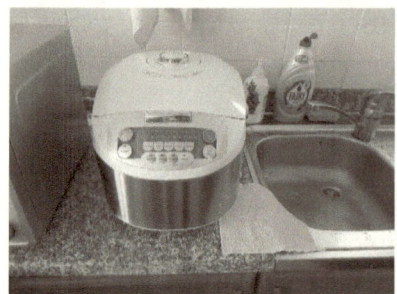
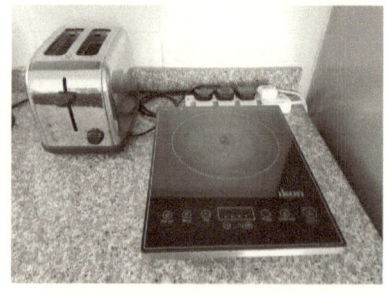
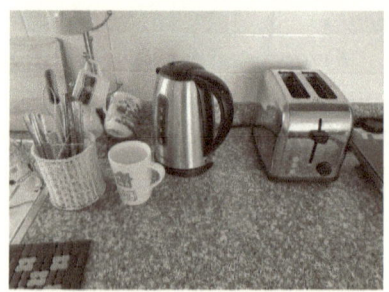

"Machines and mechanisms" for your kitchen :)

Conclusion

Let us summarize what we learn at the end of this small book:

-Diet should be safe for you and save your body;

-All successful diets relies on strong self management and regular control;

-To achieve the best result in the diet for burn your fat, - on daily basis you should receive less energy (Kcall) then spend (received Kcall < spent Kcall);

-Follow the diet should be as easy and natural as possible;

-When in pursuance of the diet - it should be treated as a way to become better and better. Yeas, you getting better and better mentally and physical in comparing to another people;

-Diet is good but usually temporarily. In order to be always in good shape you should maintain good nutrition habits;

-Nearly all medicines for speed up fat burning process have temporary effect. They work for some time and after everything return back to it's previous state. The best way to look slim and feel nice is to maintain proper nutrition habits. Right food in right time and in right quantities!

Eat healthy food, keep proper nutrition habits, respect your health and live happy long life!

Good luck!

Useful links

For those, who want to learn more about scientific or practical approach to diets and understand their body better – there some interesting links to such resources. I recommend you to follow and check them in order to have more customized approach to your healthy life

1. Professor Seluyanov (Селуянов Виктор Николаевич)
https://ru.wikipedia.org/wiki/%D0%A1%D0%B5%D0%BB%D1%83%D1%8F%D0%BD%D0%BE%D0%B2,_%D0%92%D0%B8%D0%BA%D1%82%D0%BE%D1%80_%D0%9D%D0%B8%D0%BA%D0%BE%D0%BB%D0%B0%D0%B5%D0%B2%D0%B8%D1%87

http://sportwiki.to/%D0%A1%D0%B5%D0%BB%D1%83%D1%8F%D0%BD%D0%BE%D0%B2_%D0%92%D0%B8%D0%BA%D1%82%D0%BE%D1%80_%D0%9D%D0%B8%D0%BA%D0%BE%D0%BB%D0%B0%D0%B5%D0%B2%D0%B8%D1%87

https://www.youtube.com/watch?v=BYgYkLdOmAk

Reputable and respected by many athletes scientist. Scientific approach to sport activities, bodybuilding and diets.

2. Denis Borisov
Blogs and YouTube channel (Денис Борисов)
https://fit4life.ru/
https://www.fit4life.ru/
https://24smi.org/celebrity/48288-denis-borisov.html

Reputable and respected by many athletes trainer, blogger and teacher

3. SportWiki – source of different interesting information related to bodybuilding, sport, diets and healthy life
http://sportwiki.to/%D0%AD%D0%BD
%D1%86%D0%B8%D0%BA%D0%BB%D0%BE
%D0%BF%D0%B5%D0%B4%D0%B8%D1%8F_
%D0%B1%D0%BE
%D0%B4%D0%B8%D0%B1%D0%B8%D0%BB
%D0%B4%D0%B8%D0%BD%D0%B3%D0%B0

4. Athletic Blog. Humans anatomical atlases
http://www.athleticblog.ru/
http://www.athleticblog.ru/?page_id=1081

Lot's of useful information regarding sport activities

5. Cooking Catalog
https://1000.menu/cooking

Thousands of cooking recipes. Tasty, useful, interesting and healthy

Additional materials

Energy in Kcall in a food
(please see next pages)

CALORIE VALUE OF FOOD ITEMS

(Figures given in this chart are based on 100 gm portions)

Food	Calories	Protein (gms)	Fat (gms)	Carbohydrate (gms)	Water (gms)	Vitamins
Milk	65	3.3	4	5	87	A, B$_2$, Niacin
Butter	740	-	82	-	15	A
Cream	210	2	21	3	72	A
Cheese	310	22	25	-	44	A, B$_2$, Niacin
Ice Cream	170	4	7	25	64	B$_1$, B$_2$, Niacin
Margarine	740	-	81	-	16	A
Eggs	150	12	11	-	75	A, B$_1$, B$_2$, Niacin
Pork (Grilled)	340	29	24	-	36	B$_2$, Niacin
Chicken (Roast)	150	25	5	-	55	
Fish (eg. Cod)	220	20	10	8	60	B$_1$,Niacin
Beans (Boiled)	20	2	-	3	90	A
Cabbage (Boiled)	10	1	-	1	96	A, C
Carrot (Boiled)	20	0.6	-	4	91	A
Cauliflower (Boiled)	10	1.5	-	1	93	C
Cucumber (Raw)	10	0.6	-	2	96	C
Peas (Boiled)	50	5	-	8	80	A, B$_1$, B$_2$, Niacin, C
Potatoes (Boiled)	80	1	-	22	77	B$_1$
Tomatoes	15	1	-	3	93	A, C
Apples	45	0.3	-	12	84	-
Bananas	80	1	-	20	70	C
Cherries	50	0.6	-	12	81	-
Grapes	60	0.6	-	15	80	C
Oranges	35	1	-	9	86	C, A
Pea Nuts (Roasted)	570	24	49	9	4	B$_1$, B$_2$, Niacin
Beer	30	0.3	-	2	-	-
Wine	70	-	-	-	-	-
Spirits	220	-	-	-	-	-
Coffe (Black)	-	-	-	-	-	Niacin
Bread	230	8	2	50	39	B$_1$, Nia
Rice (White Boiled)	120	2	-	30	70	-
Cornflakes with milk	205	6.5	4	34.7	-	A$_1$, B$_1$, B$_2$, Niacin, B
Chocolate Biscuits	520	6	28	67	2	B$_2$, Niacin
Wheat Bran	200	14	6	23	8	B$_1$, B$_2$, Niacin

The calorie chart of Indian food, so keep a track of the calorie intake and adopt healthy eating habits.

Calories in Fruits per 100 Grams
Calories in Apple 56
Calories in Avocado Pear 190
Calories in Banana 95
Calories in Chickoo 94
Calories in Cherries 70
Calories in Dates 281
Calories in Grapes Black 45
Calories in Guava 66
Calories in Kiwi Fruit 45
Calories in Lychies 61
Calories in Mangoes 70
Calories in Orange 53
Calories in Orange juice 100ml 47
Calories in Papaya 32
Calories in Peach 50
Calories in Pears 51
Calories in Pineapple 46
Calories in Plums 56
Calories in Strawberries 77
Calories in Watermelon 26
Calories in Pomegranate 77

Calories in Vegetables per 100 Grams
Calories in Broccoli 25
Calories in Brinjal 24
Calories in Cabbage 45
Calories in Carrot 48
Calories in Cauliflower 30
Calories in Fenugreek (Methi) 49
Calories in French beans 26
Calories in Lettuce 21
Calories in Mushroom 18
Calories in Onion 50
Calories in Peas 93
Calories in Potato 97
Calories in Spinach 100g
Calories in Spinach 1 leaf
Calories in Tomato 21
Calories in Tomato juice 100ml 22
Calories in Cereals per 100 Grams
Calories in Bajra 360
Calories in Maize flour 355
Calories in Rice 325
Calories in Wheat flour 341

Calories in Breads per piece
1 medium chapatti 119
1 slice white bread 60
1 paratha (no filling) 280

Calories in Milk & Milk Products per cup
Calories in Butter 100gms. 750
Calories in Buttermilk 19
Calories in Cheese 315
Calories in Cream 100gms. 210
Calories in Ghee 100gms 910
Calories in Milk Buffalo 115
Calories in Milk Cow 100
Calories in Milk Skimmed 45
Calories in Other Items
Calories in Sugar 1 tbsp 48
Calories in Honey 1 tbsp 90
Calories in Coconut water 100 ml 25
Calories in Coffee 40
Calories in Tea 30

The calorie chart as per U.S standards.

Apple	2.75" diameter	80
Apple juice	1 cup	115
Applesauce	1 cup unsweetened	105
Apricot	3 medium	50
Avocado	1 medium	305
Banana	1 large	105
Blueberries	1 cup	80
Cantaloupe	half of 5" diameter	95
Cherries	1cup	90
Dates	10	230
Grapefruit	half	40
Grapes, green	1 cup	90
Honeydew	6.5" wedge	45
Kiwi	1	45
Mango	4 ounces	75
Nectarine	1	75
Orange	1 medium	70
Orange juice	1 cup	105

Papaya	4 ounces	45
Peach	1 medium	50
Pear	1	100
Pineapple	8 ounces	60
Pineapple juice	4 ounces	60
Plum	1	30
Prunes	2 ounces	130
Raisins	.25 cup	120
Raspberries	1 cup	70
Strawberries	1 cup	55
Tangerine	1 medium	37
Watermelon	4" x 8" wedge	155

Vegetables

Artichoke	1 medium	50
Asparagus	4 ounces	20
Beets	4 ounces	35
Beet greens	1 cup	25
Broccoli	4 ounces	30
Brussel sprouts	1 cup	50
Cabbage, raw	1 cup	25
Carrot	1	30
Cauliflower, raw	1 cup	30
Celery	1 stalk	5
Collard greens	1 cup	25
Corn, on cob	1 ear	85
Corn, kernels	1 cup	165
Cucumber	8"	15
Dandelion	4 ounces	50
Eggplant	1 cup	25
Endive/Escarole	1 cup	10
Green beans	4 ounces	40
Kale, raw	1 cup	40

Leeks	.5 cup	16
Lettuce, head	1 cup	15
Lettuce, romaine	4 ounces	25
Mushrooms	.5 cup	9
Okra	1 cup	50
Onions, green	6 small	25
Onions, white, raw	4 ounces	40
Parsnips	1 cup	95
Peas	1 cup	125
Pepper, sweet green	1 medium	20
Pepper, sweet red	1 medium	25
Potato baked	4 ounces	125
Potato chips	10	105
Potato, french fried	6	100
Potato, mashed	.5 cup	90
Potato salad	1 cup	360
Potato, sweet	5 ounces	200
Pumpkin	1 cup	50
Radishes	4 small	8
Sauerkraut	1 cup	45
Spinach	1 cup	10
Squash, summer	.5 cup	55
Squash, winter	.5 cup	45
Squash, zucchini	1 cup	40
Tomato	1 medium	20
Turnips	1 cup	55
Turnip greens	1 cup	45
Watercress	4 ounces	25

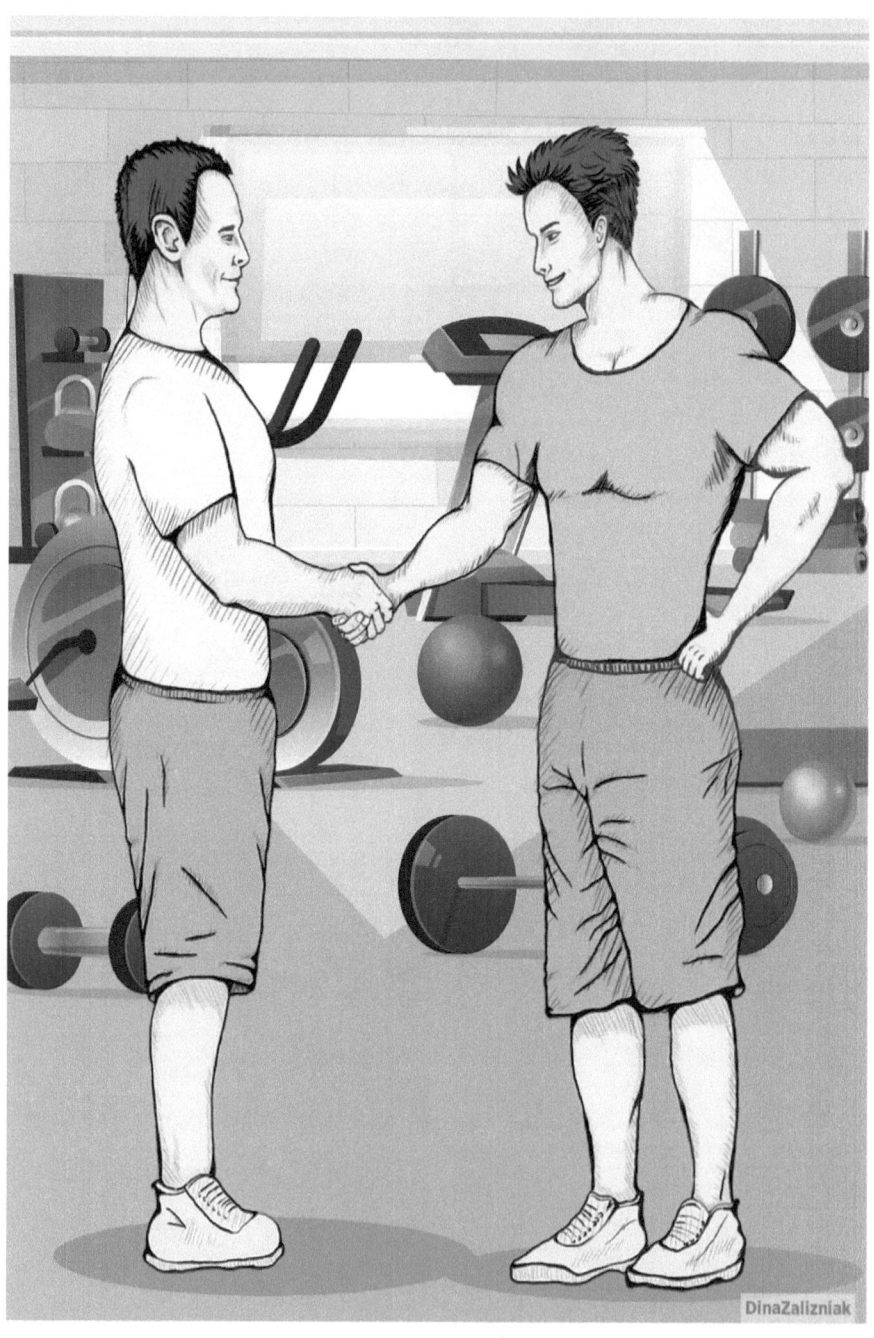

www.ingramcontent.com/pod-product-compliance
Lightning Source LLC
Chambersburg PA
CBHW050354290526
45785CB00006B/2764